The Ultimate Guide to Grocery Shopping

The Ultimate Guide to Grocery Shopping

The Ultimate Guide to Grocery Shopping

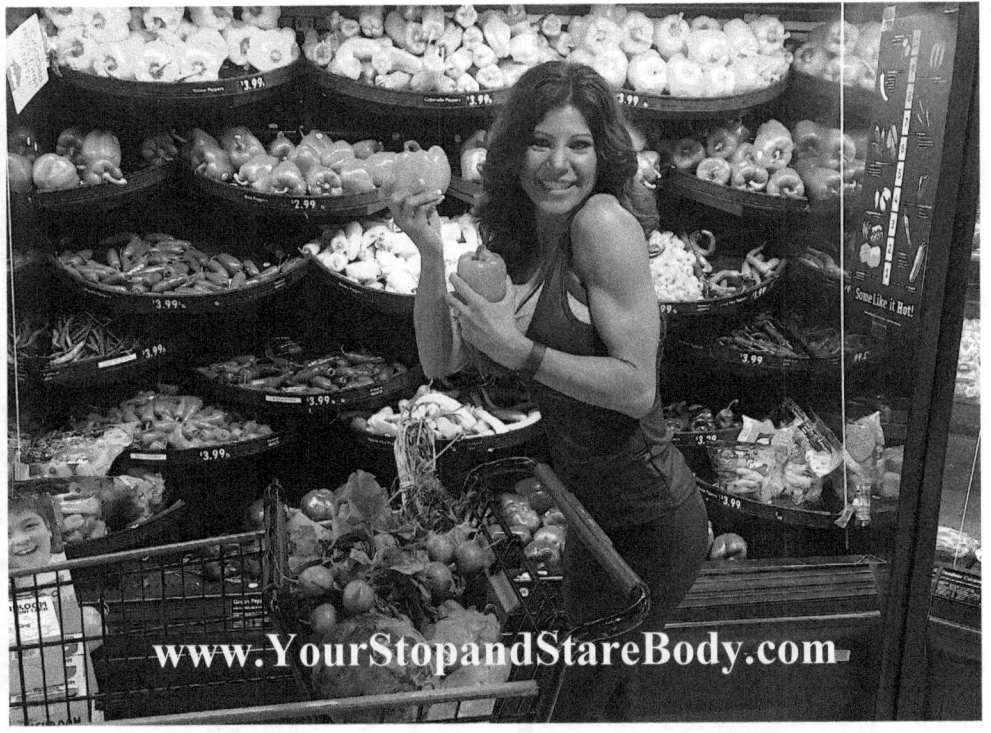

www.YourStopandStareBody.com

NEVER second-guess yourself when Grocery Shopping for your family again!

Grace Gillespie

The Ultimate Guide to Grocery Shopping

If You Keep Good Food In Your Fridge, You Will Eat Good Food

It is soooooo hard to go grocery Shopping and figure out how to buy Healthy food for your family, right? WRONG!!

Let me tell you about one of my divine passions ~ it is to help YOU make "healthy living" a lifestyle and not just a fad, learn how to read labels and make healthy choices and healthy living YOUR LIVESTYLE!

The more we invest healthy in our body, the better our ROI (return on investment) will be. ☺

Believe me, I love food just as much as anyone, but if you can take your favorite meal, alter it a little and make it healthy AND delicious, then you can have your (sugar free ;)) cake and eat it too!

I would LOVE to hear your feedback, what you thought of my book, what else you would be interested in learning about and even how this book impacted you and your families lives!!

Email me at;

YourStopandStareBody@gmail.com

Check out my other books "Your Stop and Stare Body" Mental Motivation, and my Healthy Recipe Book in the "Your Stop and Stare Body Series, to start living that healthy lifestyle and be on you way to YOUR STOP AND STARE BODY! ;)

~ Grace ☺

A Healthy Outside Starts From The Inside

Table
of
Contents

Don't Ask why Healthy Food is so Expensive...

Ask why Junk Food is so Cheap

Just the Facts

1.

Wouldn't you love to have someone go grocery shopping with you and tell you exactly what to get, why you should get it, how much you need, what exactly to make for the whole week AND how to read labels?? Weeelllll, ask and you shall receive ~ because, that's exactly what I'm going to do! I'm gonna explain all about labels, shopping, and the importance of preplanning and especially how to not only make it a habit, but make it a lifestyle!

Did you know that 80% of what you look like is what you eat?! Crazy, huh? But so true. The other 20% is how you live your life, activity level and what you do in the gym.

So doesn't it just make sense to start at the grocery store? Good nutrition starts with good choices and how can you make healthy meals if ya don't have the right ingredients in your kitchen?!
There are so many choices, false advertisements (fat free, sugar free) and hard to understand labels, that it makes

it difficult AND time consuming for the average person to be certain they're
making the right decision.

You can't believe what the advertisements, commercials and stores say, because they are hoping you buy (and eat) more food not less. So, a little knowledge can go a long way with making healthy choices and learning the best, smartest and healthiest ways to shop.

What?! Isn't everyone in Love with their Veggies?!

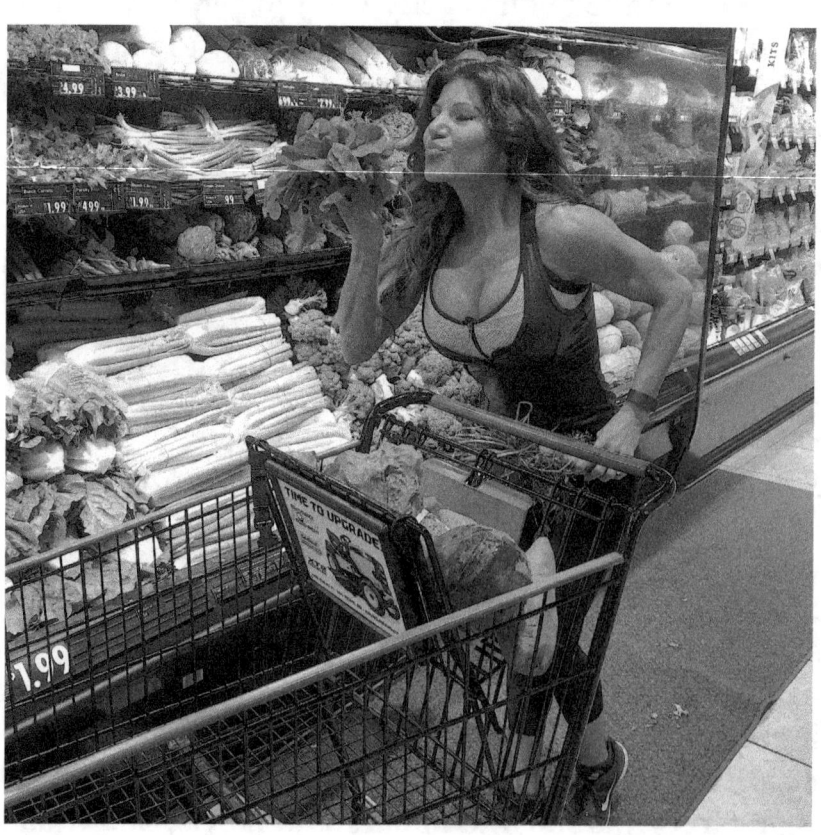

It's NOT that I CAN'T eat that... I'm making the healthier choice not to

No Sugar-Free Coating

2.

According to studies, Americans eat around 49,000 extra calories every year which translates into a grand total of 14 extra pounds of body fat per year. This is why an estimated 65% of Americans are considered to be overweight.

In essence, Americans are slowly getting fatter and it is largely from the consumption of "fat free" foods! So, the problem is ~ while "fat free" foods contain almost no actual fat, (per serving- don't forget!!) many of them DO contain high amounts of sugar. (The same goes with "Sugar free", it usually contains high amounts of fat! Vicious cycle!) It's all this SUGAR that been added to these products that allows them to be called "fat free". Consuming high amounts of sugar will (obviously) cause you to gain weight because sugar makes your blood sugar levels rise rapidly, causing a large insulin response. Insulin, particularly in high amounts, will transport much of this sugar right to your fat cells for storage.

Soooo… what can you do to prevent yourself from being lured into the labeling web of deceit?!!

Here are some things that will help clear up the blurriness of label reading so you can have a more clear view of what's really in there.

To start… ALWAYS read EVERYTHING on the label. You don't just wanna look at the fat content then only skim down at the rest. Look at the sugar content then compare it to the overall carbohydrate content to see how much of the carbohydrates are actually sugar. ALWAYS compare the calories from fat to the total calories. Fat should NOT be higher than 30% of the total calories at the absolute most!!

Next, look at the protein content and try to make sure there is at least a decent amount of it in the item. Protein rich foods like granola make good, healthy snacks.

It is also important is to look for the fiber content of certain foods. When you buy breakfast cereal for example, make sure it has at least 5 grams of dietary fiber per serving. Try to buy whole grain items like whole wheat bread and whole wheat pasta as these also provide decent amounts of fiber.

Aside from reading the labels, you should also read the list of ingredients. Here is where you get to see what is actually in each item. When buying any flour items such as bread or pasta, avoid anything with the words enriched, bleached, or white flour in the ingredients. The more enriched a product is, the less nutritious it is. White flour has very high sugar content and therefore is not the best choice. Look for items with whole wheat flour instead.

One thing that gets hidden in the list of ingredients that you really need to be aware of is the trans fats. These trans fats are cleverly disguised with the words "hydrogenated vegetable oil". These are oils that the manufacturer adds hydrogen to in order to transform them from their liquid form to a solid form. These fats are more dangerous by far than saturated fats and you know how bad saturated fats are. If you see the key word "hydrogenated" anywhere in the ingredients, put it down, back away slowly, then turn, run, and don't look back!

Always remember to read everything on both the nutrition label and the list of ingredients before buying an item. Never let yourself be fooled into thinking an item won't make you gain weight by the words "fat-free" so boldly displayed on the front of the package. It is this kind of deception that has been the cause of unwanted weight gain throughout the nation.

Remember, the FDA requires all food manufactures to disclose everything in their products to you, but it is ultimately up to you to read far enough to find it all.

So, the next time you go food shopping, take these tips with you and ensure yourself that you are making the right choices for you and your family.

PREPARE AND PREP

These are vital steps to your meal success. Before ya even head to the grocery store, make sure you plan your meals for the week, ALL MEALS! Not just dinners, or lunches but all three meals and snacks for the whole family. Then, make a grocery list of all of the ingredients you need to make all of the meals for the week.

Now, as you stroll up and down the isles at the supermarket filling your grocery cart with the items on your list, you are armed with EVERYTHING you need to make sure you choose your items wisely. Remember that making good, healthy choices is the very reason that you carefully and strategically put together your shopping list the night before.

> *ALWAYS remember, that when you see the words "fat free or "low fat" your brain automatically gives you the go-ahead.

Collards or Radishes ~ Hmm...the age old question ;-)

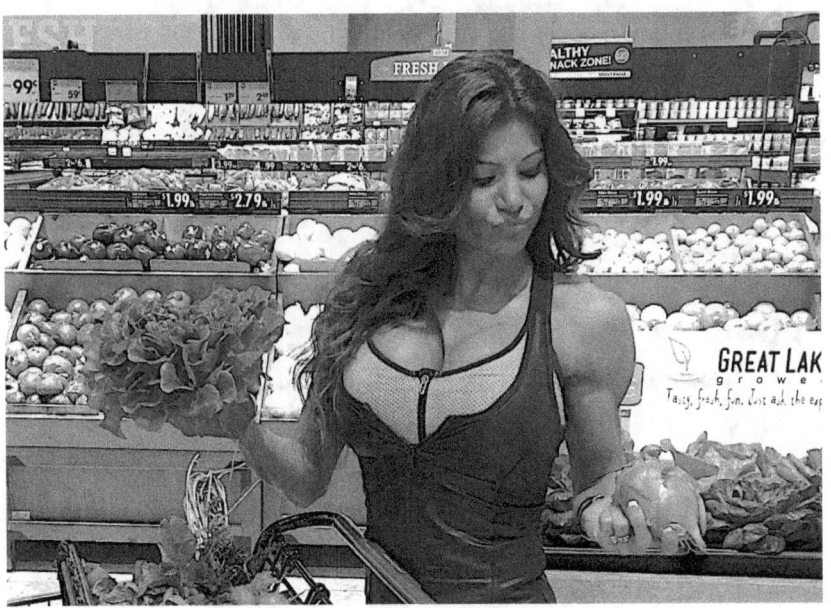

It's NEVER too Early or too Late to work towards being the Healthiest YOU!

Time to Spill the Beans

3.

WORTH THE MONEY?

Ok, so since time is money, ya need to make the decisions whether or not it is worth it to spend the extra $$$ on precut carrots, apples, single serving healthy portions, etc. If it is going to help set you up for success so you don't go crazy and throw away your portion controlling and eat junk instead of prepped carrots or grapes, then YES it is definitely worth the money! So PLEASE PLEASE keep that in mind when you're at the grocery store rushing and "hope" to have time to prepare them.

SUPERMARKET SAVVY

Use this checklist for making healthier food choices in every department of your supermarket:

PRODUCE

Spend the most time in the produce section, the first area

you encounter in most grocery stores (and usually the largest). Choose a rainbow of colorful fruits and vegetables. The colors reflect the different vitamins, minerals, and phytonutrient content of each fruit or vegetable.

BREADS, CEREALS & PASTAS

Choose the least processed foods that are made from whole grains. For example, regular oatmeal is preferable to instant oatmeal. But even instant oatmeal is a whole grain, and a good choice.

When choosing whole-grain cereals, aim for at least 4 grams of fiber per serving, and the less sugar, the better. Keep in mind that 1 level teaspoon of sugar equals 4 grams and let this guide your selections. Now, those cereals -- even those with added sugar -- make great vehicles for milk, yogurt, and/or fruit. Be cautious of granolas, even the low-fat variety; they tend to have more fat and sugar than other cereals.

Bread, pasta, rice, and grains offer more opportunities to work whole grains into your diet. Choose whole-wheat or whole grain bread and pastas, brown rice, grain mixes, quinoa, bulgur, and barley.
To help your family get used to whole grains, you can start out with whole-wheat blends and slowly transition to 100% whole-wheat /grain pasta and breads.

MEAT, FISH & POULTRY

The American Heart Association ❤ recommends two servings of fish a week. People like salmon and it's widely available, affordable, not too fishy, and a good source of omega-3 fatty acids. Be sure to choose lean cuts of meat (like round, top sirloin, and tenderloin), opt for skinless poultry, and watch your portion sizes.

DAIRY

Dairy foods are an excellent source of bone-building calcium and vitamin D. There are plenty of low-fat and nonfat options to help you get three servings a day, including drinkable and single-serve tube yogurts, and pre-portioned cheeses. If you enjoy higher-fat cheeses, no problem -- just keep your portions small.

FROZEN FOOD

Frozen fruits and vegetables (without sauce) are a convenient way to help fill in the produce gap, especially in winter. Some frozen favorites include whole-grain waffles for snacks or meals, portion-controlled bagels, 100% juices for marinades and beverages, and plain cheese pizza.

CANNED & DRIED FOODS

Keep a variety of canned vegetables, fruits, and beans on hand to toss into soups, salads, pasta, or rice dishes. Whenever possible, choose vegetables without added salt, and fruit packed in 100% real juice.

Tuna packed in water, low-fat/low sodium soups, nut butters, olive and coconut oils, and assorted vinegars should be in every healthy pantry.

A Healthy Lifestyle not only changes your Body, It changes your mind, your attitude AND your Mood!

Label Reading in the Raw

4.

SERVING SIZES
Nutrition labels tell you how many nutrients are in that serving size of food. Serving sizes help people understand how much they're eating.
Below is a description of how to read a food label, using the label of macaroni and cheese.

The information in the main or top section (see #1-4 and #6 on the sample nutrition label below) can vary with each food product; it contains product-specific information (serving size, calories, and nutrient information). The bottom part (see #5 on the sample label below) contains a footnote with Daily Values (DVs) for 2,000 and 2,500 calorie diets. This footnote provides recommended dietary information for important nutrients, including fats, sodium and fiber. The footnote is found only on larger packages and does not change from product to product.

In the following Nutrition Facts label, there are colored certain sections to help you focus on those areas that will be explained in detail. You will not see these colors on the food labels on products you purchase.

Lol... But... oh so true!

Nutrition Facts
Serving Size 1 Burger (2 if still hungry)

Amount Per Serving

Calories At this point it doesn't matter

% Daily Value

Total Fat A joke compared to the breakfast burrito I had this morning	37%
Cholesterol My medication keeps this in balance	25%
Sodium Salt releases flavor, everybody knows that	26%
Carbohydrates This is how I get my videogame energy	10%
Protein Under these rolls it's all muscle	

Self-control 0%	Ketchup on shirt 16%
Perspiration 60%	Happiness 24%

Sample Label for Macaroni and Cheese

Nutrition Facts

Serving Size 1 cup (228g)
Servings Per Container 2

(1) **Start Here** ➡

Amount Per Serving

Calories 250   Calories from Fat 110

(2) **Check Calories**

	% Daily Value*
Total Fat 12g	18%
Saturated Fat 3g	15%
Trans Fat 3g	
Cholesterol 30mg	10%
Sodium 470mg	20%
Total Carbohydrate 31g	10%

(3) **Limit these Nutrients**

(6) **Quick Guide to % DV**

Dietary Fiber 0g	0%
Sugars 5g	
Protein 5g	
Vitamin A	4%
Vitamin C	2%
Calcium	20%
Iron	4%

• **5% or less is Low**

• **20% or more is High**

(4) **Get Enough of these Nutrients**

* Percent Daily Values are based on a 2,000 calorie diet.
Your Daily Values may be higher or lower depending on
your calorie needs.

	Calories	2,000	2,500
Total Fat	Less than	65g	80g
Sat Fat	Less than	20g	25g
Cholesterol	Less than	300mg	300mg
Sodium	Less than	2,400mg	2,400mg
Total Carbohydrate		300g	375g
Dietary Fiber		25g	30g

(5) **Footnote**

(Info provided by FDA.gov)

1. THE SERVING SIZE

(#1 on sample label)
Serving Size section of label.

The first place to start when you look at the Nutrition Facts label is the serving size and the number of servings in the package. Serving sizes are standardized to make it easier to compare similar foods; they are provided in familiar units, such as cups or pieces, followed by the metric amount, e.g., the number of grams.

The size of the serving on the food package influences the number of calories and all of the nutrient amounts listed on the top part of the label. Pay attention to the serving size, especially how many servings there are in the food package. Then ask yourself, "How many servings am I consuming"? (e.g., 1/2 serving, 1 serving, or more) In the sample label, one serving of macaroni and cheese equals one cup. If you ate the whole package, you would eat two cups. That doubles the calories and other nutrient numbers, including the %Daily Values as shown in the sample label.

Example					
	Single Serving	%DV		**Double Serving**	%DV
Serving Size	1 cup (228g)			2 cups (456g)	
Calories	250			500	
Calories from Fat	110			220	
Total Fat	12g	18%		24g	36%
Trans Fat	1.5g			3g	
Saturated Fat	3g	15%		6g	30%
Cholesterol	30mg	10%		60mg	20%
Sodium	470mg	20%		940mg	40%
Total Carbohydrate	31g	10%		62g	20%
Dietary Fiber	0g	0%		0g	0%
Sugars	5g			10g	
Protein	5g			10g	
Vitamin A		4%			8%
Vitamin C		2%			4%
Calcium		20%			40%
Iron		4%			8%

***Learning how to read labels will save you from eating tons of unwanted calories!**

2. CALORIES (AND CALORIES FROM FAT)

Calories provide a measure of how much energy you get from a serving of this food. Many Americans consume more calories than they need without meeting recommended intakes for a number of nutrients. The calorie section of the label can help you manage your weight (i.e., gain, lose, or maintain.)
Remember: the number of servings you consume determines the number of calories you actually eat (your portion amount).

(#2 on sample label)

Calories from Fat section of label, also showing total calories.

In the example, there are 250 calories in one serving of this macaroni and cheese. How many calories from fat are there in ONE serving? Answer: 110 calories, which means almost half the calories in a single serving come from fat. What if you ate the whole package content? Then, you would consume two servings, or 500 calories, and 220 would come from fat.

General Guide to Calories

~ 40 Calories is low
~ 100 Calories is moderate
~ 400 Calories or more is high

The General Guide to Calories provides a general reference for calories when you look at a Nutrition Facts label. This guide is based on a 2,000 calorie diet.

*Eating too many calories per day is linked to overweight and obesity.

3 AND 4. THE NUTRIENTS: HOW MUCH?

Look at the top of the nutrient section in the sample label. It shows you some key nutrients that impact on your health and separates them into two main groups:
*LIMIT THESE NUTRIENTS

(#3 on sample label) Label section showing Total Fat, Saturated Fat, Cholesterol, and Sodium, with quantities and % daily values.

Total Fat 12g	18%
Saturated Fat 3g	15%
Trans Fat 3g	
Cholesterol 30mg	10%
Sodium 470mg	20%

The nutrients listed first are the ones Americans generally eat in adequate amounts, or even too much. They are identified in yellow as Limit these Nutrients. Eating too much fat, saturated fat, trans fat, cholesterol, or sodium may increase your risk of certain chronic diseases, like heart disease, some cancers, or high blood pressure.

*Important: Health experts recommend that you keep your intake of saturated fat, trans fat and cholesterol as low as possible as part of a nutritionally balanced diet.

Get Enough of These

Dietary Fiber 0g	0%
Vitamin A	4%
Vitamin C	2%
Calcium	20%
Iron	4%

(#4 on sample label)
Label sections showing Dietary Fiber, Vitamin A, Vitamin C, Calcium, and Iron, with % daily values and quantity of dietary fiber.

Most Americans don't get enough dietary fiber, vitamin A, vitamin C, calcium, and iron in their diets. They are identified in blue. Eating enough of these nutrients can improve your health and help reduce the risk of some diseases and conditions. For example, getting enough calcium may reduce the risk of osteoporosis, a condition that results in brittle bones as one ages. (see calcium section below) Eating a diet high in dietary fiber promotes healthy bowel function. Additionally, a diet rich in fruits, vegetables, and grain products that contain dietary fiber, particularly soluble fiber, and low in saturated fat and cholesterol may reduce the risk of heart disease.

Remember: You can use the Nutrition Facts label not only to help limit those nutrients you want to cut back on but also to increase those nutrients you need to consume in greater amounts.

5. UNDERSTANDING THE FOOTNOTE ON THE BOTTOM OF THE NUTRITION FACTS LABEL

(#5 on sample label)
Foootnote section of label, indicating values for 2000 and 2500 calorie diets highlighting the statement: *

		Calories:	2,000	2,500
*Percent Daily Values are based on a 2,000 calorie diet. Your Daily Values may be higher or lower depending on your calorie needs.				
Total Fat	Less than		65g	80g
Sat Fat	Less than		20g	25g
Cholesterol	Less than		300mg	300mg
Sodium	Less than		2,400mg	2,400mg
Total Carbohydrate			300g	375g
Dietary Fiber			25g	30g

Percent Daily Values are based on a 2000 calorie diet.

Note the * used after the heading "%Daily Value" on the Nutrition Facts label. It refers to the Footnote in the lower part of the nutrition label, which tells you "%DVs are based on a 2,000 calorie diet". This statement must be on all food labels. But the remaining information in the full footnote may not be on the package if the size of the label is too small. When the full footnote does appear, it will always be the same. It doesn't change from product to product, because it shows recommended dietary advice for all Americans--it is not about a specific food product.

Look at the amounts circled in the footnote--these are the Daily Values (DV) for each nutrient listed and are based on public health experts' advice. DVs are recommended levels of intakes. DVs in the footnote are based on a 2,000 or 2,500 calorie diet. Note how the DVs for some nutrients change, while others (for cholesterol and sodium) remain the same for both calorie amounts.

Do It For The AFTER Selfie ;)

A Grain of Sea Salt

5.

HOW THE DAILY VALUES RELATE TO THE %DVS

Look at the example below for another way to see how the Daily Values (DVs) relate to the %DVs and dietary guidance. For each nutrient listed there is a DV, a %DV, and dietary advice or a goal. If you follow this dietary advice, you will stay within public health experts' recommended upper or lower limits for the nutrients listed, based on a 2,000 calorie daily diet.

Examples of DVs versus %DVs

Based on a 2,000 Calorie Diet

Nutrient	DV	%DV	Goal
Total Fat	65g	= 100%DV	Less than
Sat Fat	20g	= 100%DV	Less than
Cholesterol	300mg	= 100%DV	Less than
Sodium	2400mg	= 100%DV	Less than
Total Carbohydrate	300g	= 100%DV	At least
Dietary Fiber	25g	= 100%DV	At least

UPPER LIMIT - EAT "LESS THAN"...

The nutrients that have "upper daily limits" are listed first on the footnote of larger labels and on the example above. Upper limits means it is recommended that you stay below - eat "less than" - the Daily Value nutrient amounts listed per day. For example, the DV for Saturated fat (in the yellow section) is 20g. This amount is 100% DV for this nutrient. What is the goal or dietary advice? To eat "less than" 20 g or 100%DV for the day.<

LOWER LIMIT - EAT "AT LEAST"...

Now look at the section in blue where dietary fiber is listed. The DV for dietary fiber is 25g, which is 100% DV. This means it is recommended that you eat "at least" this amount of dietary fiber per day.

The DV for Total Carbohydrate (section in white) is 300g or 100%DV. This amount is recommended for a balanced daily diet that is based on 2,000 calories, but can vary, depending on your daily intake of fat and protein.

Now let's look at the %DVs.

How Hard can this be? ;-)

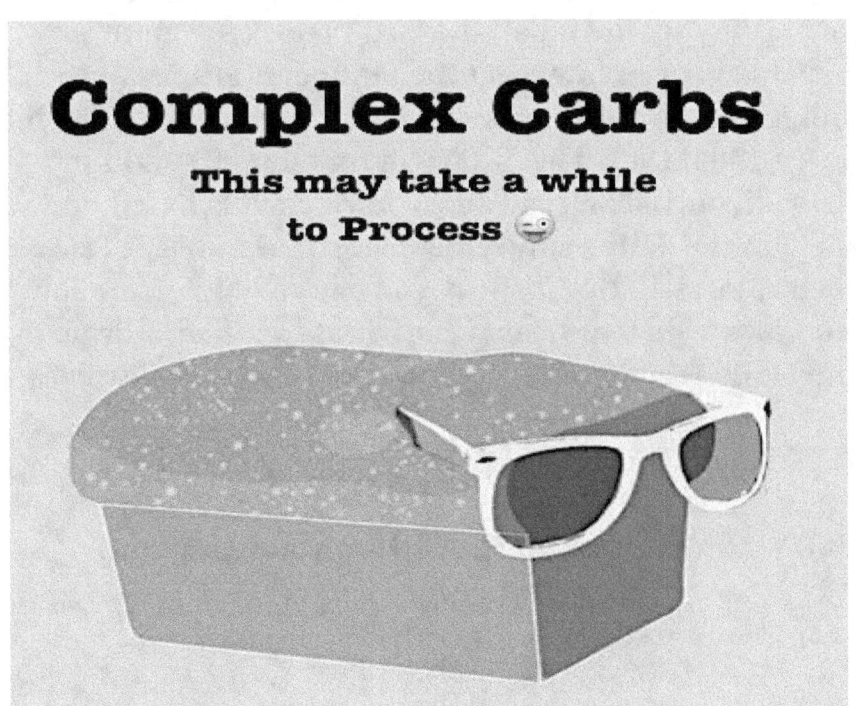

6. THE PERCENT DAILY VALUE (%DV)

The % Daily Values (%DVs) are based on the Daily Value recommendations for key nutrients but only for a 2,000 calorie daily diet--not 2,500 calories. You, like most people, may not know how many calories you consume in a day. But you can still use the %DV as a frame of reference whether or not you consume more or less than 2,000 calories.

The %DV helps you determine if a serving of food is high or low in a nutrient.

Note: a few nutrients, like trans fat, do not have a %DV--they will be discussed later.

Do you need to know how to calculate percentages to use the %DV? No, the label (the %DV) does the math for you. It helps you interpret the numbers (grams and milligrams) by putting them all on the same scale for the day (0-100%DV). The %DV column doesn't add up vertically to 100%. Instead each nutrient is based on 100% of the daily requirements for that nutrient (for a 2,000 calorie diet). This way you can tell high from low and know which nutrients contribute a lot, or a little, to your daily recommended allowance (upper or lower).

QUICK GUIDE TO %DV

5%DV or less is low and 20%DV or more is high

(#6 on sample label)

This guide tells you that 5%DV or less is low for all nutrients, those you want to limit (e.g., fat, saturated fat, cholesterol, and sodium), or for those that you want to consume in greater amounts (fiber, calcium, etc). As the Quick Guide shows, 20%DV or more is high for all nutrients.

Example: Look at the amount of Total Fat in one serving listed on the sample nutrition label. Is 18%DV contributing a lot or a little to your fat limit of 100% DV? Check the Quick Guide %DV. 18%DV, which is below 20%DV, is not yet high, but what if you ate the whole package (two servings)? You would double that amount, eating 36% of your daily allowance for Total Fat. Coming from just one food, that amount leaves you with 64% of your fat allowance (100%-36%=64%) for all of the other foods you eat that day, snacks and drinks included.

	% Daily Value*
Total Fat 12g	18%
Saturated Fat 3g	15%
Trans Fat 3g	
Cholesterol 30mg	10%
Sodium 470mg	20%
Total Carbohydrate 31g	10%
Dietary Fiber 0g	0%
Sugars 5g	
Protein 5g	
Vitamin A	4%
Vitamin C	2%
Calcium	20%
Iron	4%

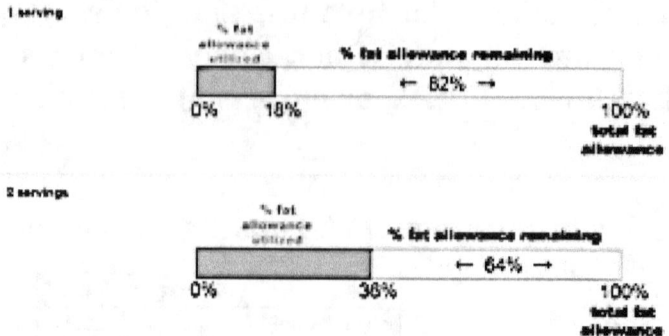

USING THE %DV

Comparisons: The %DV also makes it easy for you to make comparisons. You can compare one product or brand to a similar product. Just make sure the serving sizes are similar, especially the weight (e.g. gram, milligram, ounces) of each product. It's easy to see which foods are higher or lower in nutrients because the serving sizes are generally consistent for similar types of foods, (see the comparison example at the end) except in a few cases like cereals.

Nutrient Content Claims: Use the %DV to help you quickly distinguish one claim from another, such as "reduced fat" vs. "light" or "nonfat." Just compare the %DVs for Total Fat in each food product to see which one is higher or lower in that nutrient--there is no need to memorize definitions. This works when comparing all nutrient content claims, e.g., less, light, low, free, more, high, etc.

You Can't Expect to Look Like a Million Bucks if You Eat from the Dollar Menu

Dietary Trade-Offs: You can use the %DV to help you make dietary trade-offs with other foods throughout the day. You don't have to give up a favorite food to eat a healthy diet. When a food you like is high in fat, balance it with foods that are low in fat at other times of the day. Also, pay attention to how much you eat so that the total amount of fat for the day stays below 100%DV.

My Puppies even make Healthy Choices! ;-)

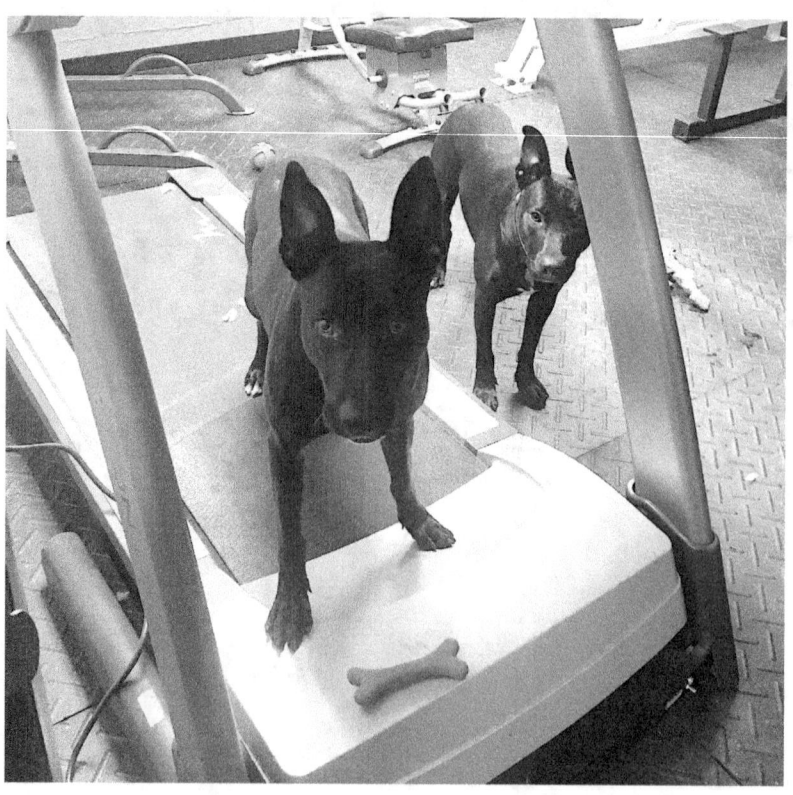

NUTRIENTS WITH A %DV BUT NO WEIGHT LISTED - SPOTLIGHT ON CALCIUM

Label of nonfat milk with calcium daily value of 30% circled.

Calcium: Look at the %DV for calcium on food packages so you know how much one serving contributes to the total amount you need per day. Remember, a food with 20%DV or more contributes a lot of calcium to your daily total, while one with 5%DV or less contributes a little.

Experts advise adult consumers to consume adequate amounts of calcium, that is, 1,000mg or 100%DV in a daily 2,000 calorie diet. This advice is often given in milligrams (mg), but the Nutrition Facts label only lists a %DV for calcium.

Nutrition Facts

Serving Size 1 cup (236ml)
Servings Per Container 1

Amount Per Serving

Calories 80   Calories from Fat 0

	% Daily Value*
Total Fat 0g	0%
Saturated Fat 0g	0%
Trans Fat 0g	
Cholesterol Less than 5mg	0%
Sodium 120mg	5%
Total Carbohydrate 11g	4%
Dietary Fiber 0g	0%
Sugars 11g	
Protein 9g	17%

Vitamin A 10% • Vitamin C 4%
Calcium 30% • Iron 0% • Vitamin D 25%

*Percent Daily Values are based on a 2,000 calorie diet. Your daily values may be higher or lower depending on your calorie needs

For certain populations, they advise that adolescents, especially girls, consume 1,300mg (130%DV) and post-menopausal women consume 1,200mg (120%DV) of calcium daily. The DV for calcium on food labels is 1,000mg.

Don't be fooled -- always check the label for calcium

because you can't make assumptions about the amount of calcium in specific food categories. Example: the amount of calcium in milk, whether skim or whole, is generally the same per serving, whereas the amount of calcium in the same size yogurt container (8oz) can vary from 20-45 %DV.

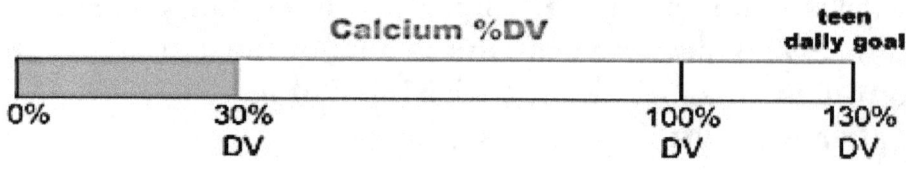

Equivalencies
30% DV = 300mg calcium = one cup of milk
100% DV = 1,000mg calcium
130% DV = 1,300mg calcium

NUTRIENTS WITHOUT A %DV: TRANS FATS, PROTEIN, AND SUGARS:
Note that Trans fat, Sugars, and protein do not list a %DV on the Nutrition Facts label.

Trans Fat: Experts could not provide a reference value for trans fat nor any other information that FDA believes is sufficient to establish a Daily Value or %DV. Scientific reports link trans fat (and saturated fat) with raising blood LDL ("bad") cholesterol levels, both of which increase your risk of coronary heart disease, a leading cause of death in the US.
IMPORTANT: HEALTH EXPERTS RECOMMEND THAT YOU KEEP YOUR INTAKE OF SATURATED

FAT, TRANS FAT AND CHOLESTEROL AS LOW AS POSSIBLE AS PART OF A NUTRITIONALLY BALANCED DIET.

Protein: A %DV is required to be listed if a claim is made for protein, such as "high in protein". Otherwise, unless the food is meant for use by infants and children under 4 years old, none is needed. Current scientific evidence indicates that protein intake is not a public health concern for adults and children over 4 years of age.

Sugars: No daily reference value has been established for sugars because no recommendations have been made for the total amount to eat in a day. Keep in mind, the sugars listed on the Nutrition Facts label include naturally occurring sugars (like those in fruit and milk) as well as those added to a food or drink. Check the ingredient list for specifics on added sugars.

Couldn't Resist!

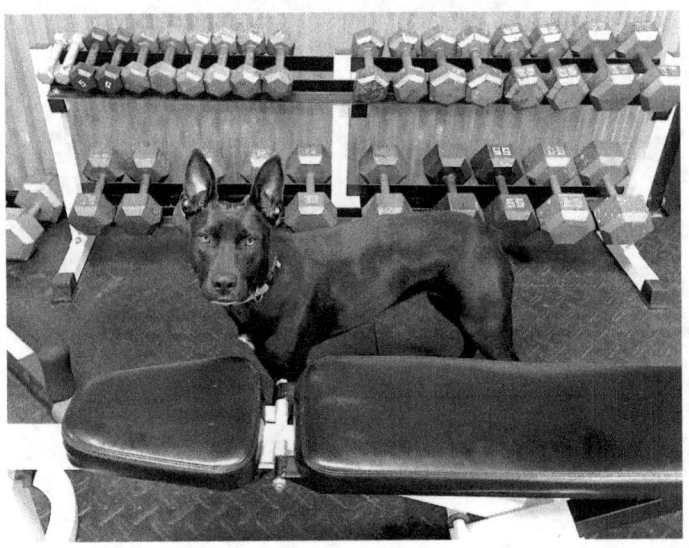

Take a look at the Nutrition Facts label for the two yogurt examples. The plain yogurt on the left has 10g of sugars, while the fruit yogurt on the right has 44g of sugars in one serving.

Now look below at the ingredient lists for the two yogurts. Ingredients are listed in descending order of weight (from most to least). Note that no added sugars or sweeteners are in the list of ingredients for the plain yogurt, yet 10g of sugars were listed on the Nutrition Facts label. This is because there are no added sugars in plain yogurt, only naturally occurring sugars (lactose in the milk).

Plain Yogurt

Nutrition Facts
Serving Size 1 container (226g)

Amount Per Serving

Calories 110 Calories from Fat 0

	% Daily Value*
Total Fat 0g	0 %
Saturated Fat 0g	0 %
Trans Fat 0g	
Cholesterol Less than 5mg	1 %
Sodium 160mg	7 %
Total Carbohydrate 15g	5 %
Dietary Fiber 0g	0 %
Sugars 10g	
Protein 13g	

Vitamin A 0 % • Vitamin C	4 %
Calcium 45 % • Iron	0 %

*Percent Daily Values are based on a 2,000 calorie diet. Your Daily Values may be higher or lower depending on your calorie needs.

Fruit Yogurt

Nutrition Facts
Serving Size 1 container (227g)

Amount Per Serving

Calories 240 Calories from Fat 25

	% Daily Value*
Total Fat 3g	4 %
Saturated Fat 1.5g	9 %
Trans Fat 0g	
Cholesterol 15mg	5 %
Sodium 140mg	6 %
Total Carbohydrate 46g	15 %
Dietary Fiber Less than 1g	3 %
Sugars 44g	
Protein 9g	

Vitamin A 2 % • Vitamin C	4 %
Calcium 35 % • Iron	0 %

*Percent Daily Values are based on a 2,000 calorie diet. Your Daily Values may be higher or lower depending on your calorie needs.

Plain Yogurt - contains no added sugars

Ingredients: Cultured pasteurized grade A nonfat milk, whey protein concentrate, pectin, carrageenan.

Fruit Yogurt - contains added sugars

Ingredients: Cultured grade A reduced fat milk, apples, high fructose corn syrup, cinnamon, nutmeg, natural flavors, and pectin. Contains active yogurt and L. acidophilus cultures.

If you are concerned about your intake of sugars, make sure that added sugars are not listed as one of the first few ingredients. Other names for added sugars include: corn syrup, high-fructose corn syrup, fruit juice concentrate, maltose, dextrose, sucrose, honey, and maple syrup.

To limit nutrients that have no %DV, like trans fat and sugars, compare the labels of similar products and choose the food with the lowest amount.

A food pyramid or diet pyramid is a pyramid-shaped diagram representing the optimal number of servings to be eaten each day from each of the basic food groups.

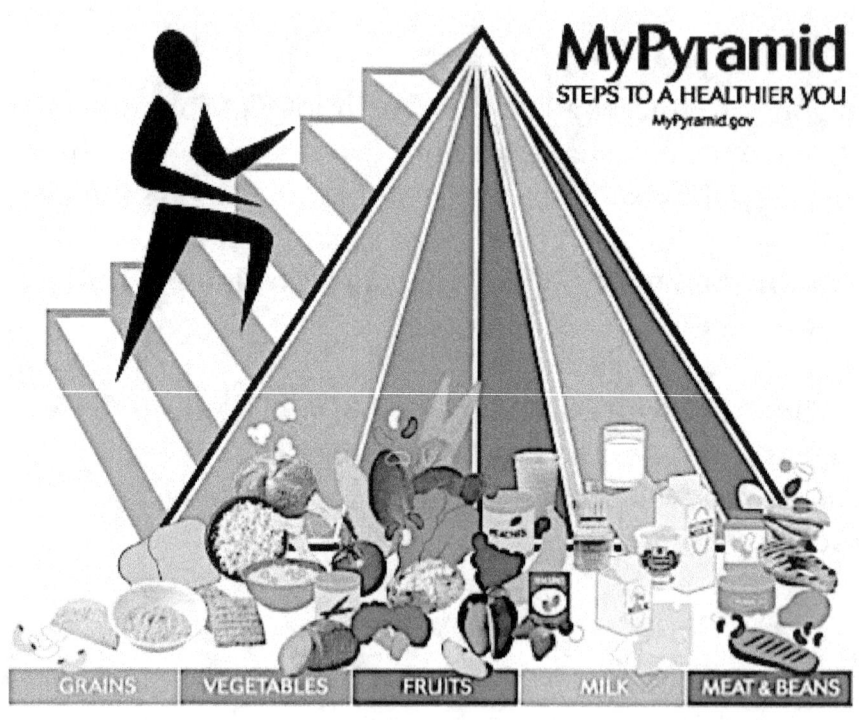

Some info was obtained from WebMD and Wikipedia.

Your Road To SUCCESS

6.

I know, I know this was a lot to take in, but I promise you, the more you review this, the more it will start to make sense! Sometimes the easiest things to do, seem to be the most difficult. But if you'll just let your Mind take the lead instead of your fork, you've already got a head start. ☺

Making Healthy a lifestyle has so many more benefits than making Healthy Living an every once in a while occurrence and trust me, the pros way outlive the cons. (Couldn't help myself , I'm in a pun kinda mood!)

Now, I've devised up a **Starter Grocery checklist for you to help you along the way (to the grocery store) and set you up for Success, so let's go… the only Road block is YOU! Let's push your old self out of the way to make room for YOUR NEW Amazing, Healthy Lifestyle, Expert Grocery Shopper, Positive Thinker YOU!! ☺**

Me LOVE me some Peppers! ;-)

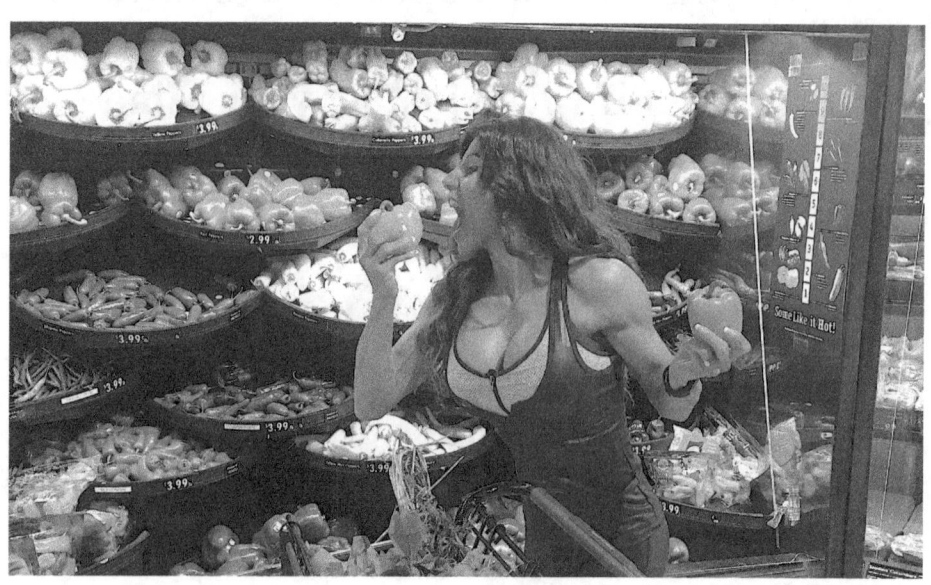

Eat Your Veggies... Have Less Wedgies!

;)

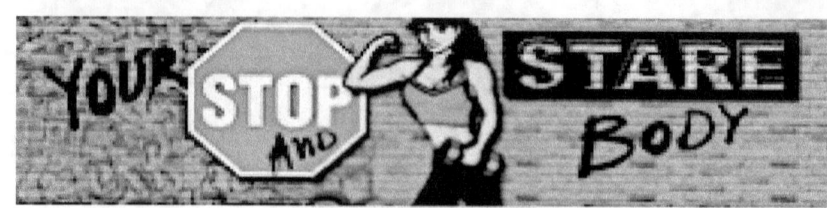

Grocery List

Produce		
Oranges		Asparagus
Apples		Broccoli
Bananas		Carrots
Grapes		Cauliflower
Tomatoes		Celery
Kiwi		Mushrooms
Avocados		Peppers
Grapefruit		Spinach
Berries		Cucumber
		Misc.
Dairy		Oatmeal
Fat Free Milk or Almond Milk		Sweet Potatoes
Low/Fat Free Cheese		Dried Fruit
Eggs		Almonds/nuts/Seeds
Cottage cheese		All Natural Peanut Butter
Low Fat Greek Yogurt		Wheat Crackers
Low Fat Yogurt		Low Sugar/Fat Protein Bars
I Can't believe its not Butter Spray		Granola
Meat		Low Salt Plain Popcorn
Extra Lean Ground Beef		Rice Cakes
Boneless/Skinless Chicken Breast		Hummus
Cod/Tilapia/Salmon/		**Oils/Spices**
Shrimp		Olive Oil
Lean Steak Cuts		Flax oil
Extra Lean Ground Turkey		Coconut Oil
Drinks		Black Pepper
PURE O.J. or fav Juice		Basil
Sparkling Soda Water		Cilantro
Coffee		Cinnamon
Tea		Garlic
Water		Ginger
Pasta/ Breads		Mint
Whole Grain/Wheat Bagels		Oregano
Whole Grain/Wheat Bread		Paprika
Whole Grain/Wheat Wraps		Red Pepper
Brown Rice		Sea Salt or Vegetable Salt
Couscous		
Quinoa		
Whole Grain/Wheat Pasta		
Frozen		
Veggie Burgers		
Sweet Potato Fries		
Veggies		
Whole Grain Waffles		
Sugar Free Popsicles		
Canned Foods		
Tuna in water		
Applesauce		
Black Kidney/Garbanzo Beans		
Olives		
Low Sodium Soups		
Misc.		
Oatmeal		
Sweet Potatoes		
Dried Fruit		
Almonds/nuts/		

That's All Folks!

7.

So there you have it! EVERYTHING you need for a successful trip to the Grocery store!   Now, you have NO excuses to come back with anything but the best for you and your family!!

My Goal is to help you reach your Goal! That means ~ I will be with you EVERY step of the way!

Visit my Websites for Daily Motivation, Tips, Articles, Health and Fitness information and Workout Videos!
www.YourStopandStareBody.com
www.FitnessByGrace.net

You now have all of the Ingredients to start living a Healthy, Happy Lifestyle, so from this point you just have to buy the ingredients and make the Recipe of Healthy Living!

Are you READY…? Then let's go Shopping!!
Good Luck and God Bless You with good healthy and Happiness ALWAYS!

Healthy isn't a Goal, It's a Way of Living

References

1. WebMD. (2016). www.webmd.com

2. Wikipedia. (2016). www.en.m.wikipedia.org

3. U.S. Food & Drug Administration. (2016). www.fda.gov

4. College Humor. (2016). www.collegehumor.com